DAILY WORKOUT GUIDE 2024

11 EASY EXERCISES VITAL FOR MEN OVER 50 YEARS TO BURN BELLY FAT AND FEEL HEALTHY.

ISRAEL H. ERHART

DISCLAIMER

All Right reserved 2024 Israel H. Erhart B. No part of this publication may be reproduced, distributed or transmitted in any form or by any means, include photocopying, recording or other electronic or mechanical methods, without the prior written permission of the publisher

TABLE

Table of Contents

ACKNOWLEDGEMENT

I would like to appreciate my Father for his motivation to do this.

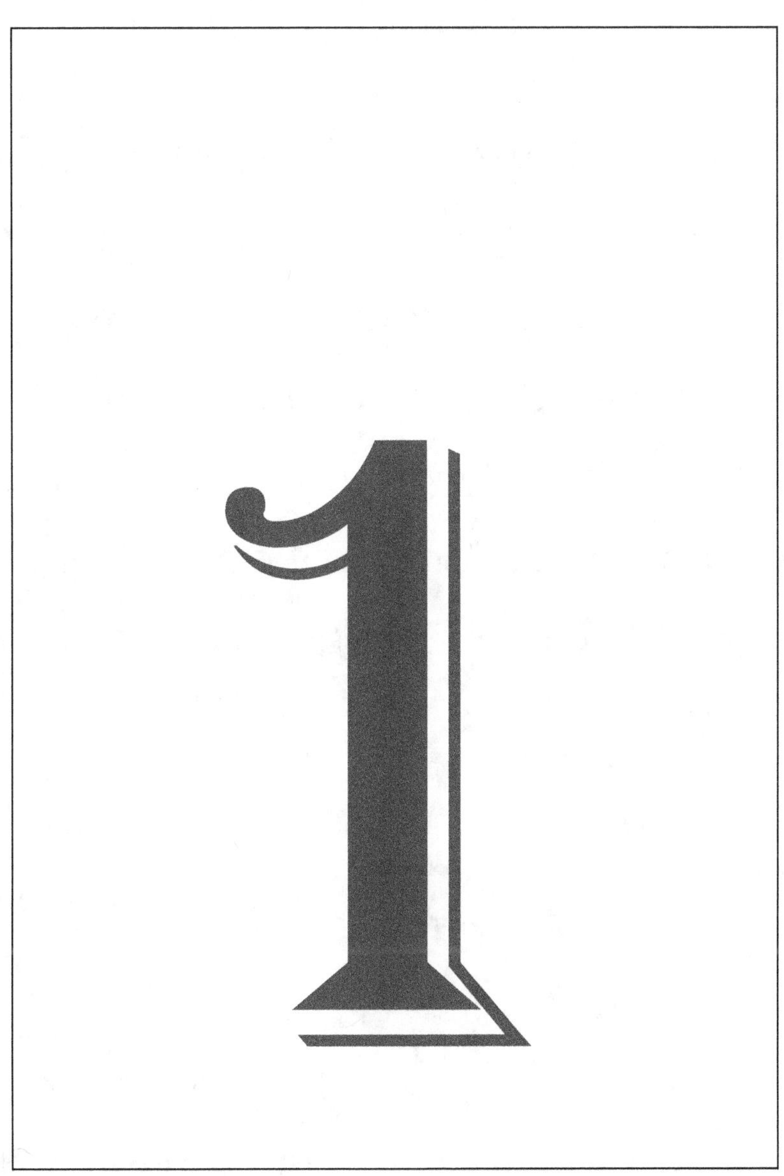

BURPEES

If you have any desire to lose your stomach, you really want to fill in whatever number muscles as could reasonably be expected. The burpee does precisely that. The unstable activity - which involves going from a push-up position to a leap and back to a push-up position - hits each muscle from head to toe.

Example

- Stand with your feet shoulder-width separated.
- Bring down your body until your palms lay on the floor about shoulder-width separated.

- Kick your legs in reverse into a push-up position, play out a push-up, and afterward rapidly switch the development and play out a leap when you stand. That is 1 rep.

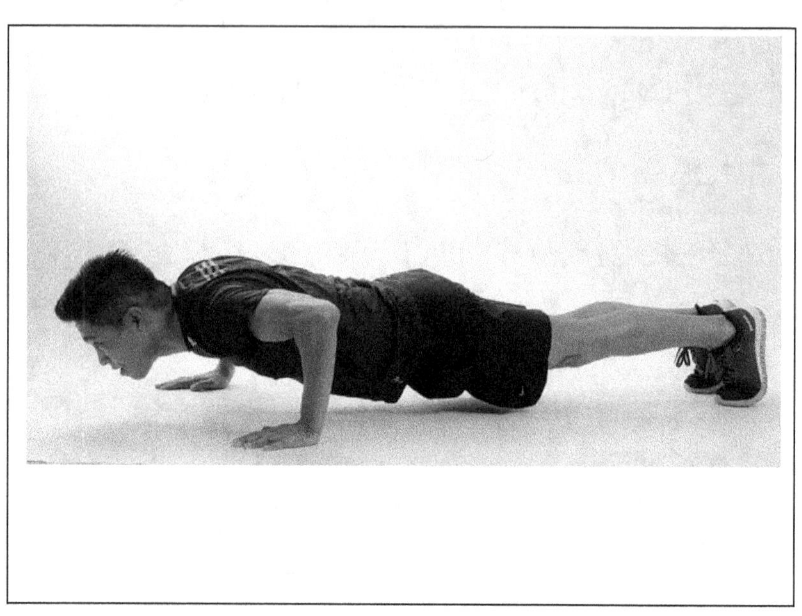

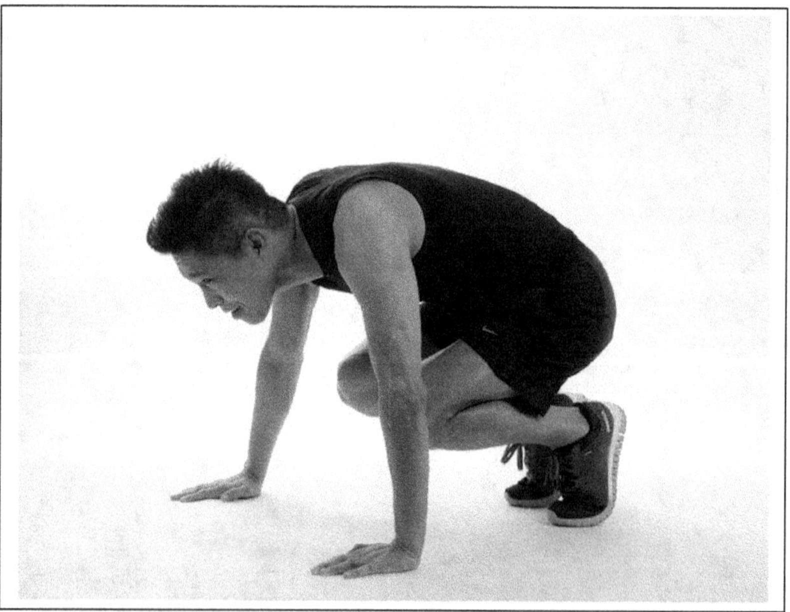

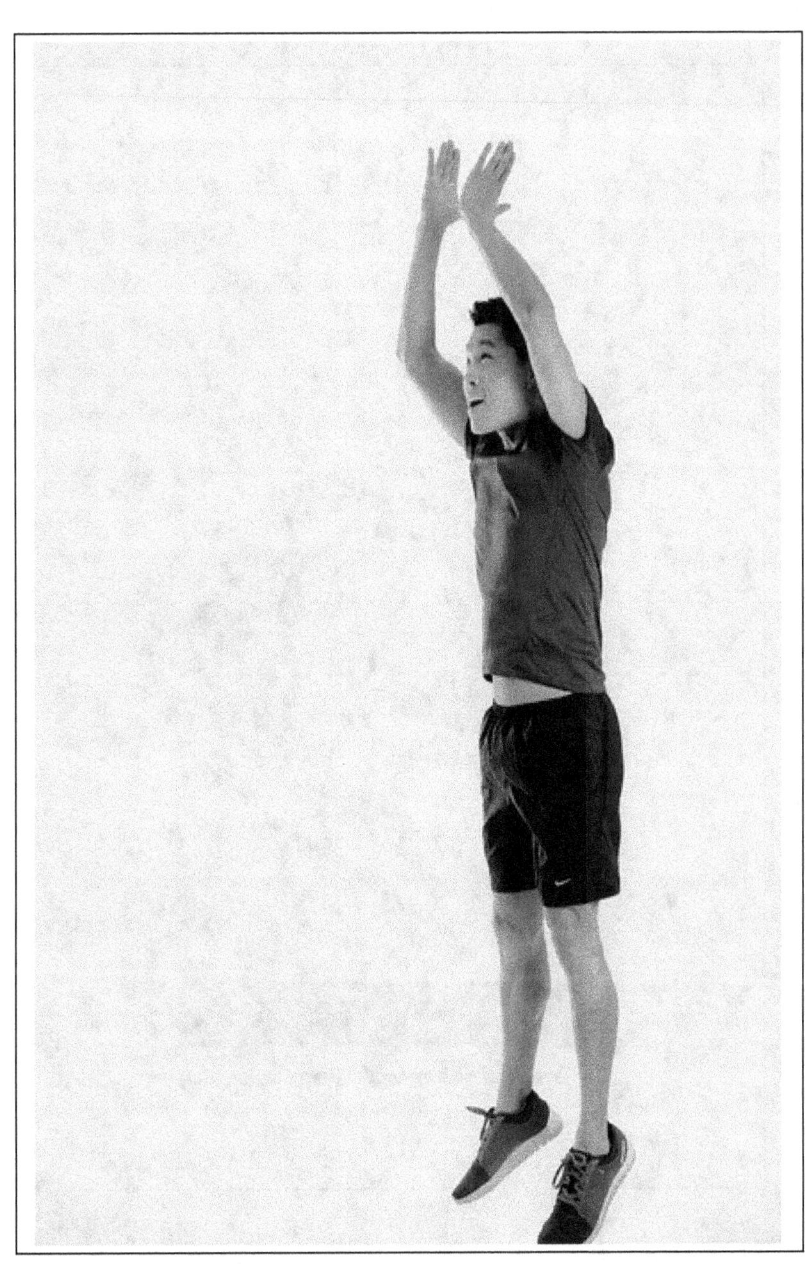

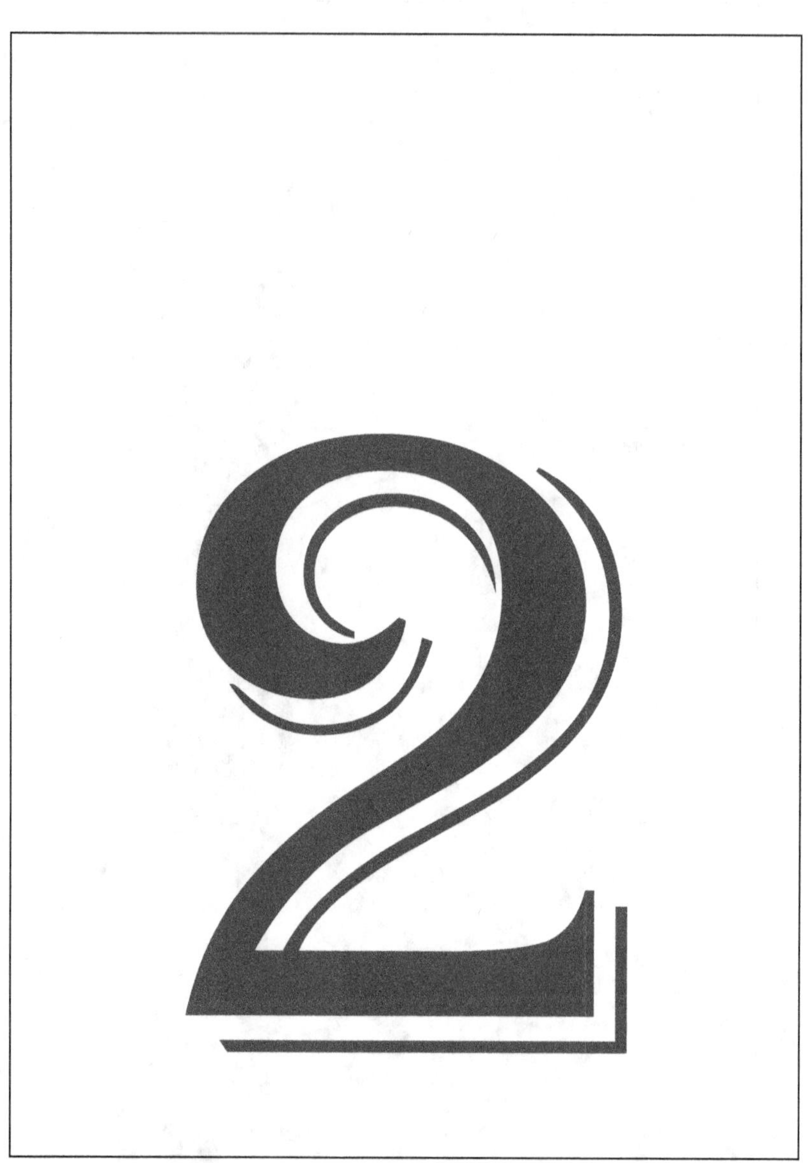

SIT UPS

Think about the Laying your back down and looking up. In some cases your legs should not shake from the floor while your upper body comes up like you are trying to sit up. What makes this activity so Intense regardless, is that it focuses on your abdomen region and your back.

Example

- Put yourself in a laying down position with your hands put behind your head like a pillow. This is the starting position.
- Now remove only your higher back from the ground, Use your hands and support your head while coming up but do not

sit erect, then go back down again

before coming back up.

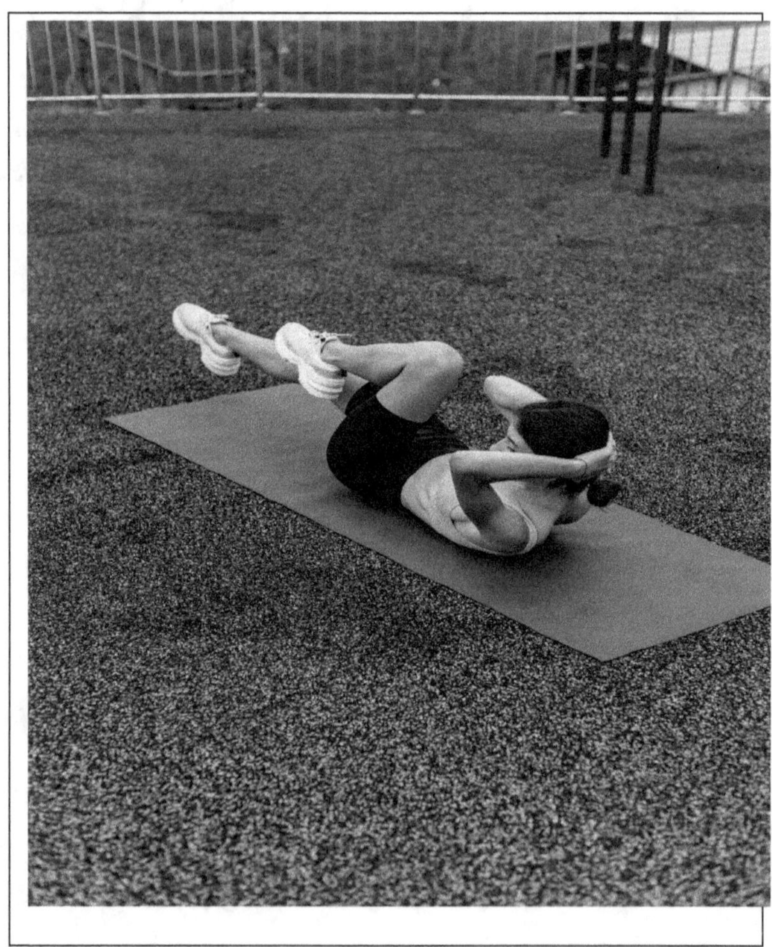

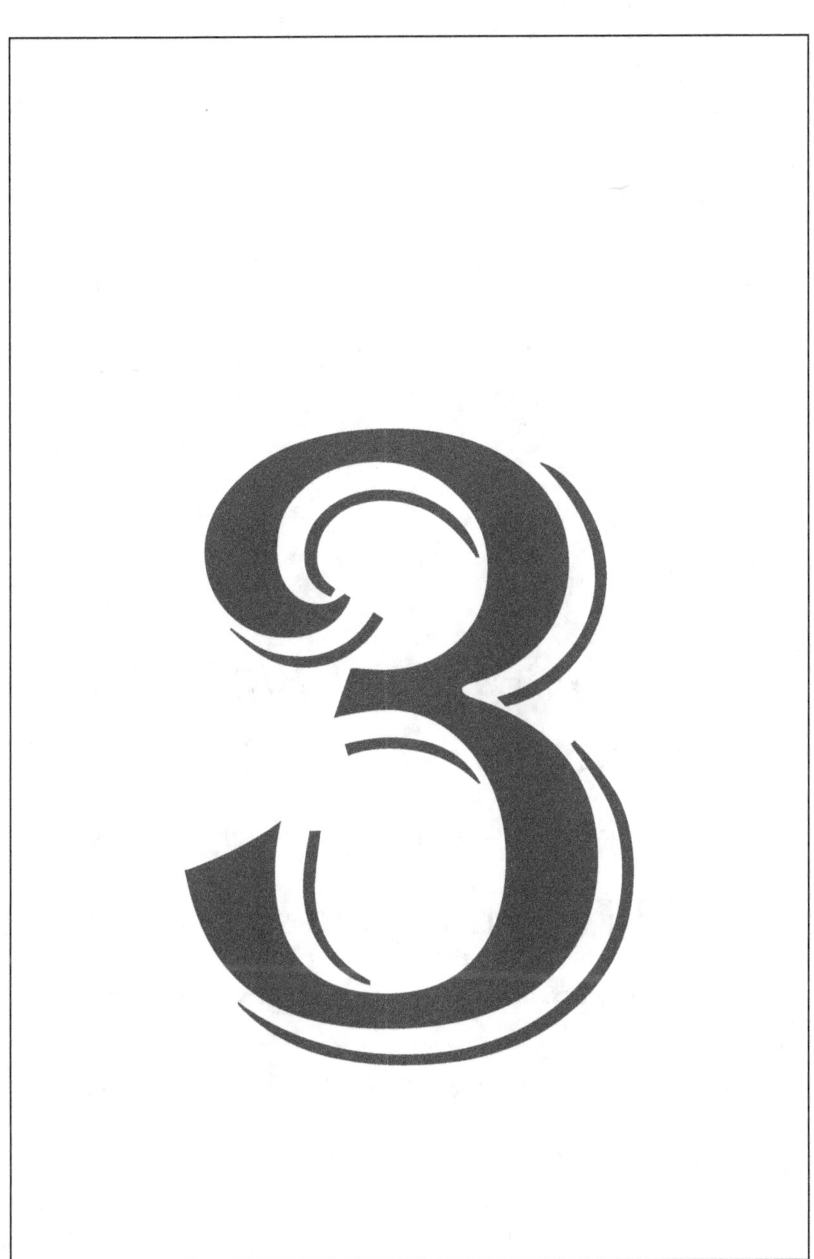

JUMPING JACKS

Jumping jacks aren't an activity saved for your half-arsed warm-up, they light calories, are great for you heart and should be possible without question, anyplace.

Example:

- Stand with your feet together and your hands at your sides. At the same time raise your arms over your head and hop up barely enough to spread your feet out wide. Without stopping.
- Immediately invert the development and rehash.

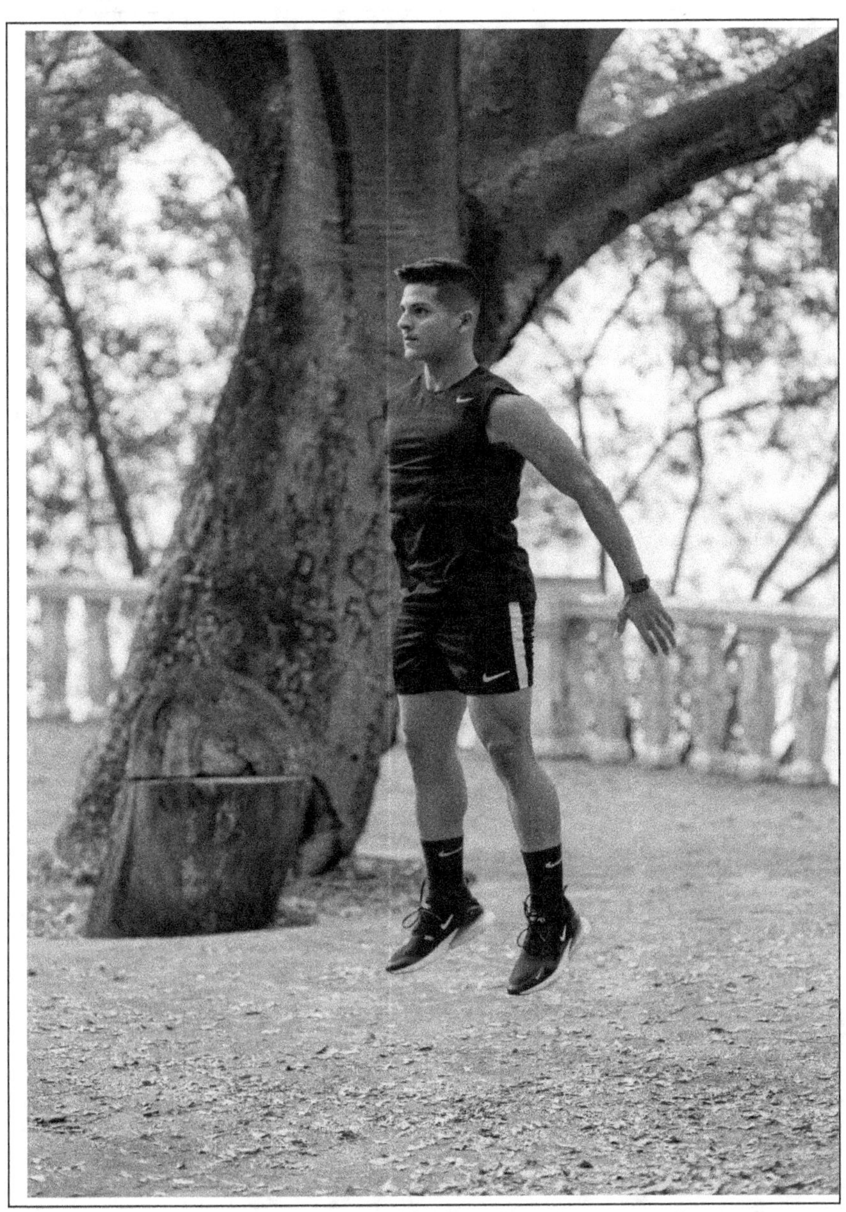

JUMPING LUNGE

Thought the free weight above rush was the main jump you want in your life? Hang on a second, a basic bouncing lurch is likewise a successful calorie executioner and, similar to that other activity, it'll work your center as well.

Example:

- Lunge forward until your back knee is practically contacting the ground.
- Hop up high, presenting your back foot forward and the front foot back. Land in a lurch and rehash.

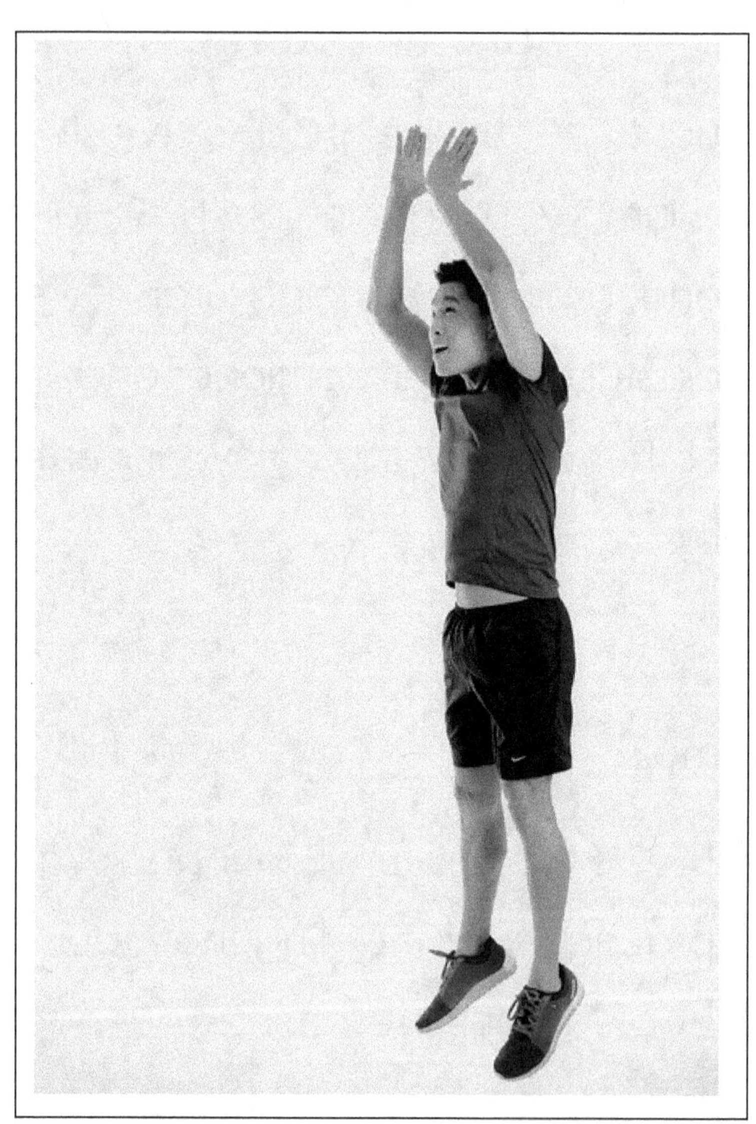

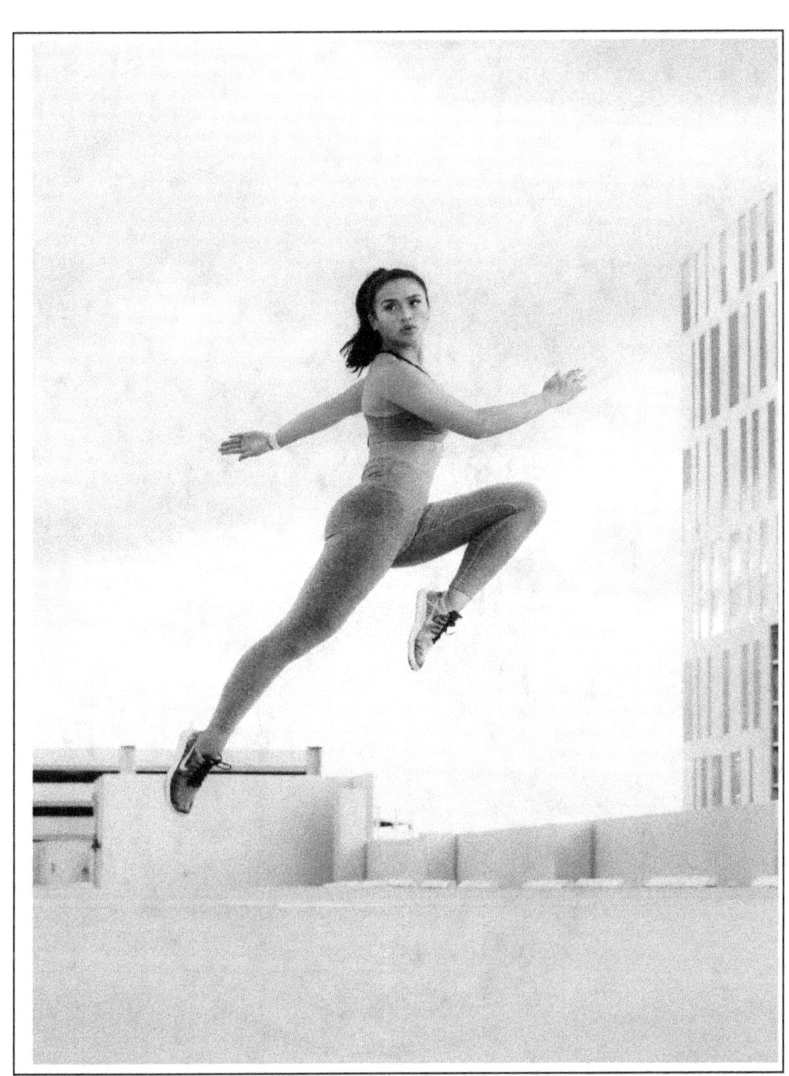

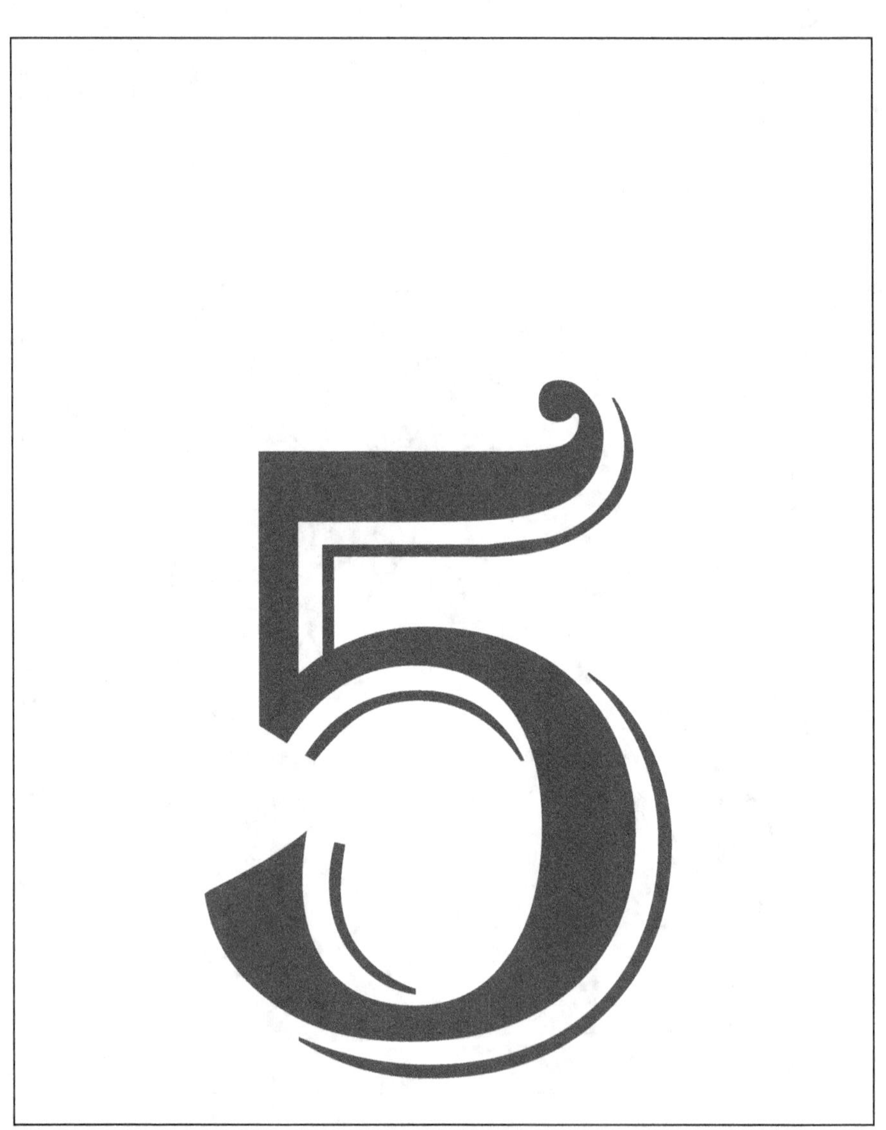

SKIPPING

Working out with rope for an hour can consume somewhere in the range of 800 and 1000 calories, and keeping in mind that we don't anticipate that you should skip for that long, don't underrate how much good a basic jumping rope can do.

Example:

- Grasp the rope with your arms by your sides.
- Hop on every upset.
- Center around keeping knees delicate and center locked in.

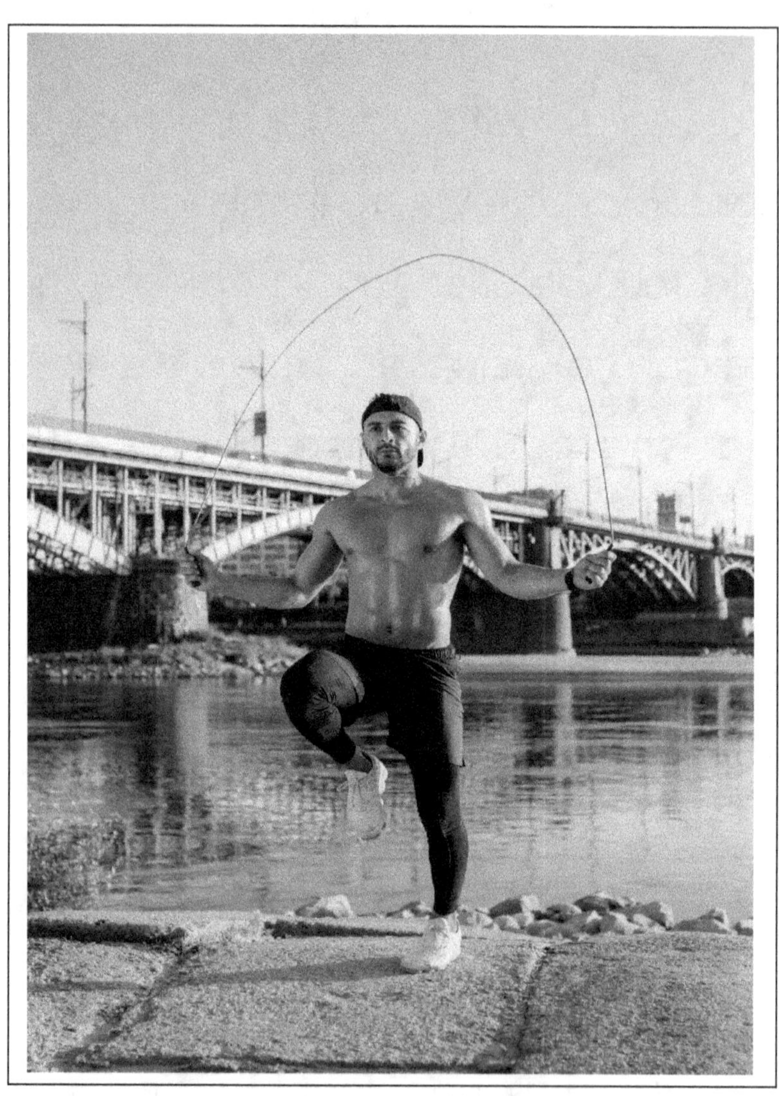

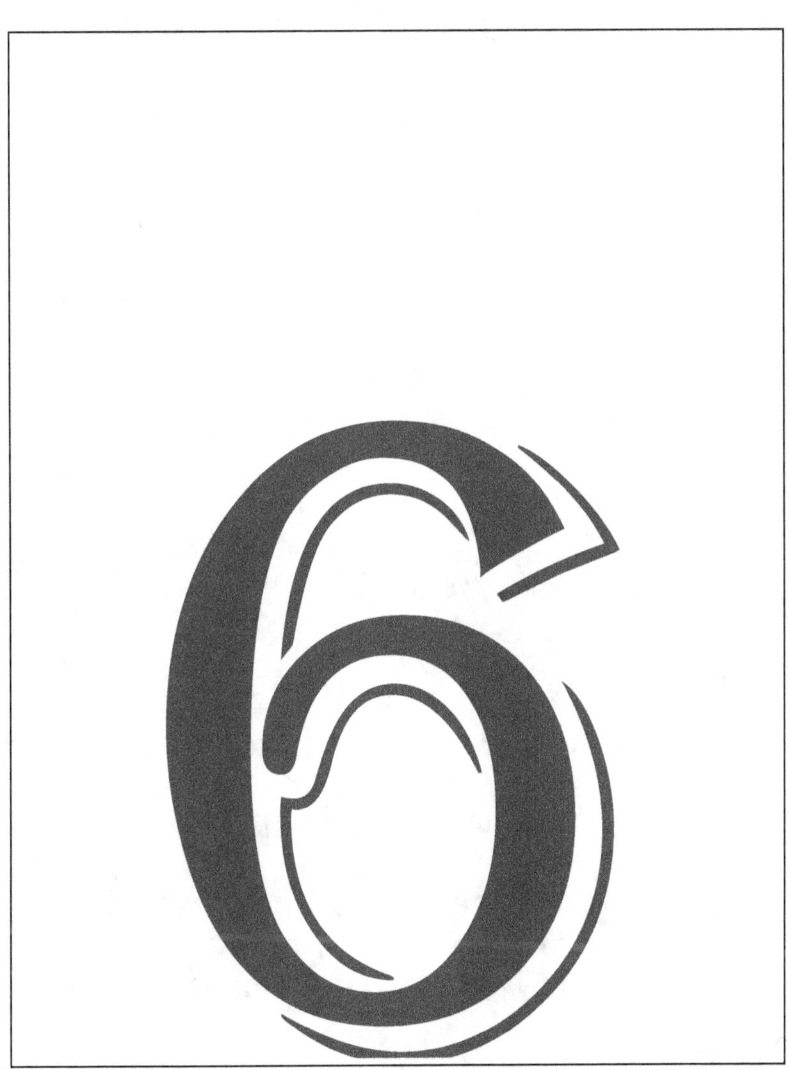

SQUAT JUMPS

Another calorie-sizzling development, squat leaps are a structure block for practically every explosive lower body development under the sun.

Example:

- Stand with your feet hip-width separated. Pivot at the hips to push your butt back and lower down until your thighs are lined up with the floor.
- Press your feet down to detonate off the floor and hop as high as possible.
  - Permit your knees to twist 45 degrees when you land, and afterward quickly

drop down into a squat, and bounce once more.

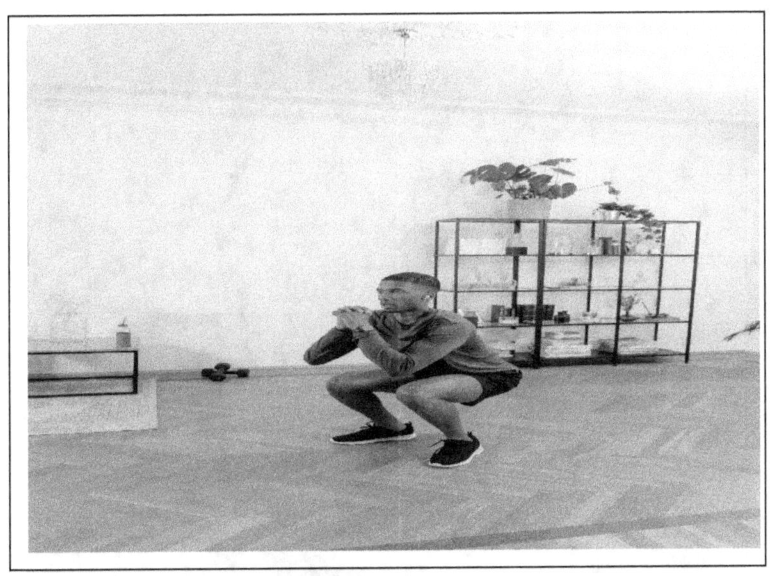

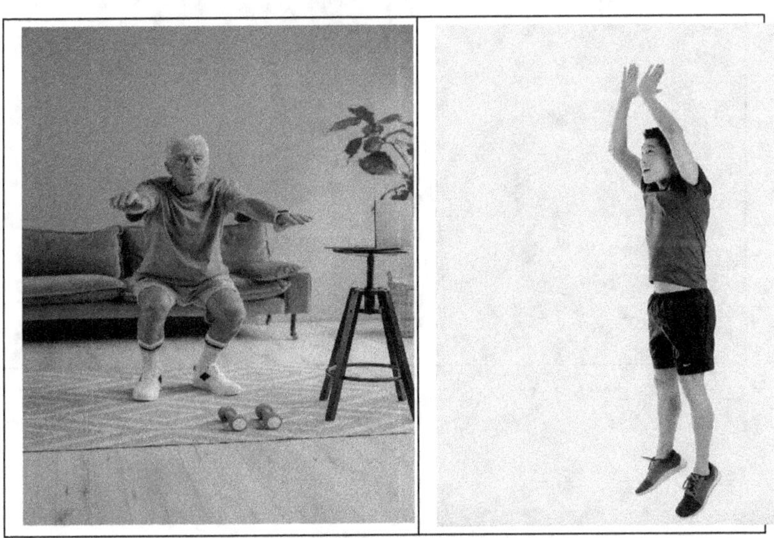

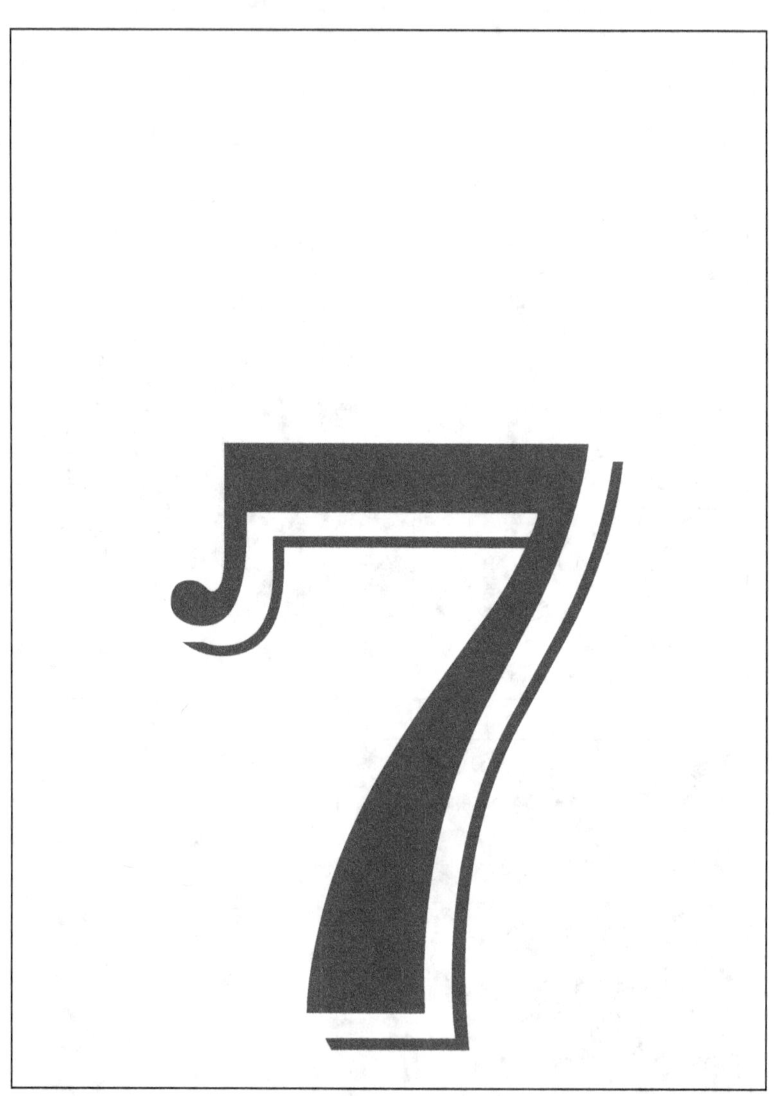

PUSH-UP

Push-up is a typical workout practice starting from the inclined position. By raising and bringing down the body utilizing the arms.

Example

- From a standard push-up position, bring down your chest until it's somewhat beneath the level of your twisted elbow, and afterward push up with sufficient power so your hands leave the ground by a couple inches.
- Land with delicate elbows in push-up structure and proceed with the bringing

down movement toward the ground.
Repeat.

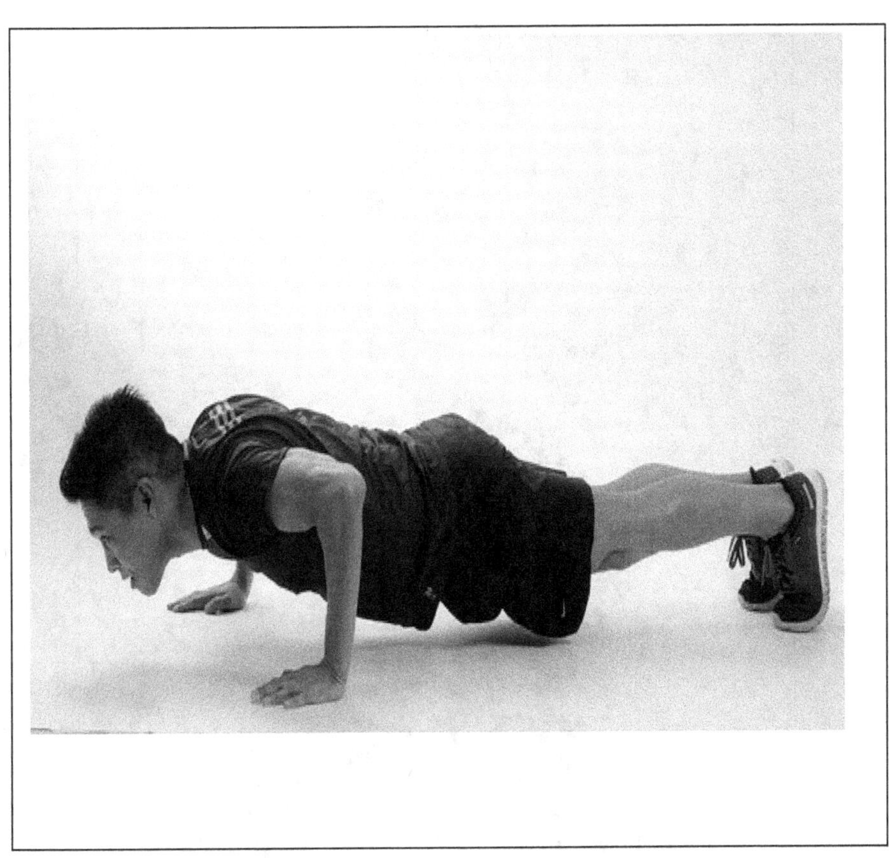

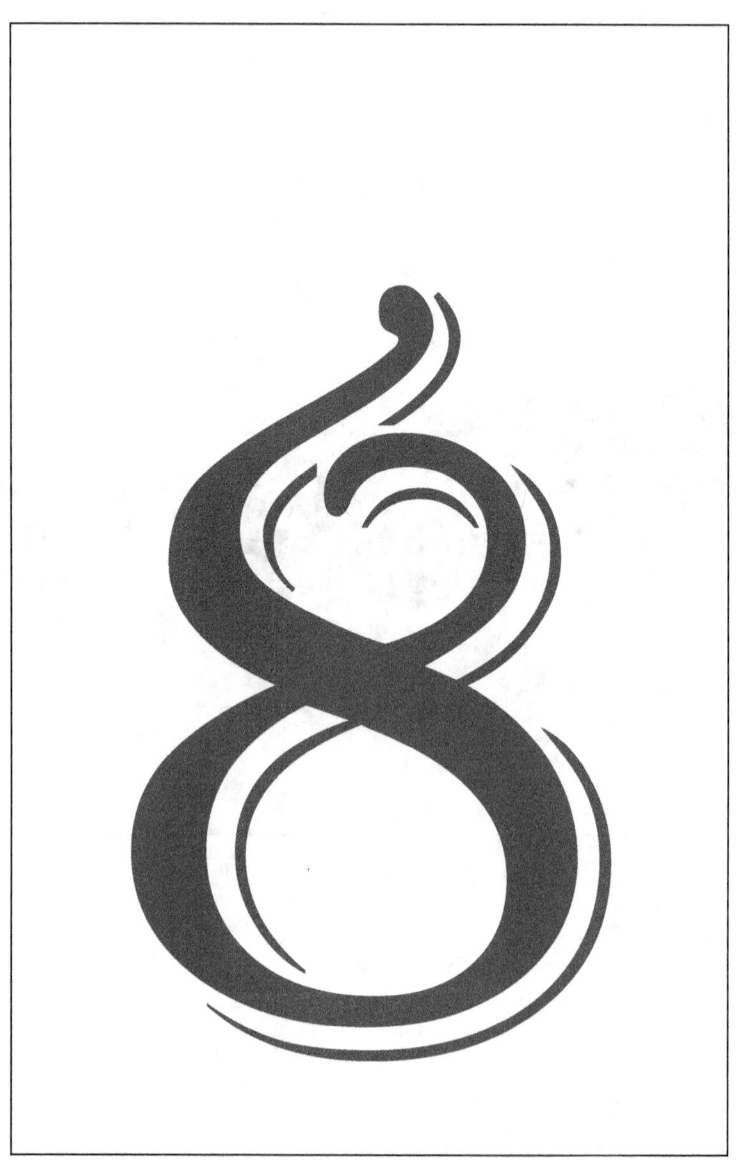

PLANKING

You'll draw in your whole center when you really do Planks the correct way. That implies your abs (abdominis rectus), the cross over abdominis, and obliques, yet additionally your low back muscles and glutes, which are critical to keeping yourself in the appropriate stance.

Example

Get all the way down. Stack your elbows straightforwardly underneath your shoulders and broaden your legs. Lay your weight on your elbows and your toes.

Crush your glutes and center to make full-body pressure. Imagine pulling your midsection button into your spine.

Contract your low back, lats, and rhomboids. Your back ought to shape a straight line; don't allow your pelvis to plunge down or your butt to ascend.

Look face down, which keeps your neck in a nonpartisan position.

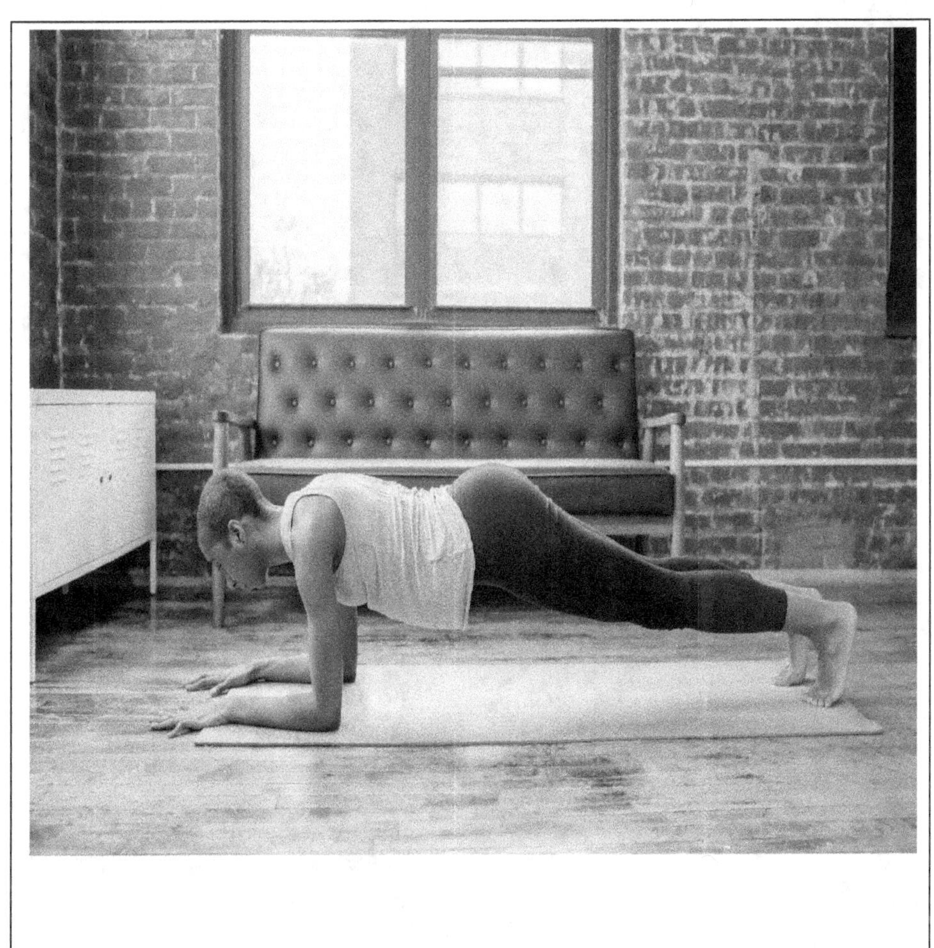

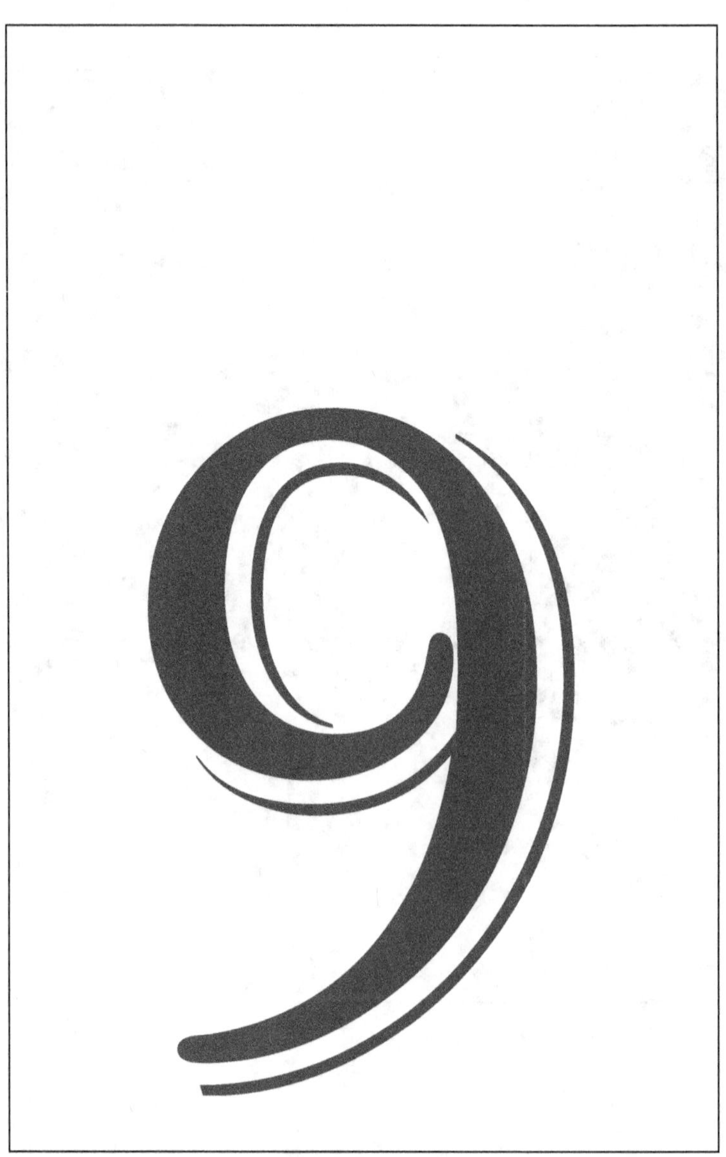

BICYCLE RIDE

Cycling is principally an aerobic action, and that implies that your heart, veins and lungs all get an exercise. You will inhale much clearer, sweat and experience extended internal heat level, which will further develop your general wellness level.

Biking is a first rate cardio exercise. You'll Release around 400 calories per 60 minutes. Additionally it reinforces your lower body, including your legs, hips, and glutes.

Assuming you need an exercise that is delicate on your back, hips, knees, and lower legs, this is a pleasant decision.

You can cycle out and about, a bicycle way, or a mountain trail.

In the event that you're a starter, pick a level bicycle way or street. Assuming you're prepared for a harder exercise that likewise connects with your chest area and center, attempt mountain Biking. It's additionally canceled street trekking. You can do it on trails and various kinds of harsh territory.

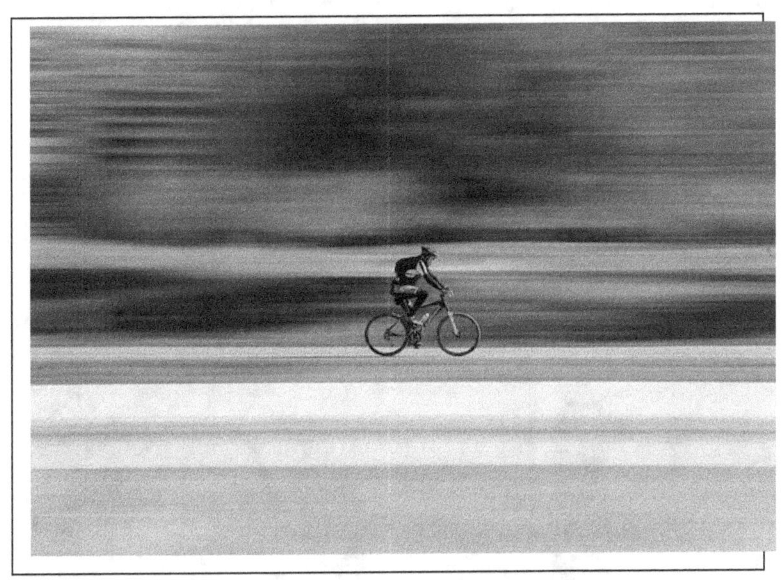

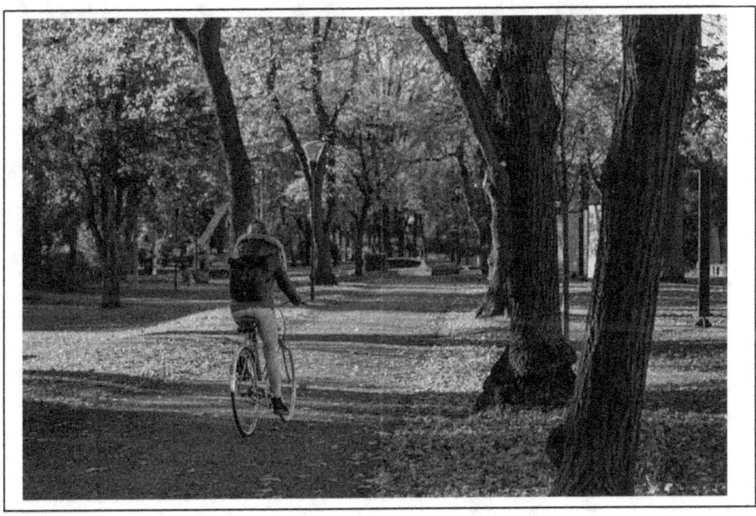

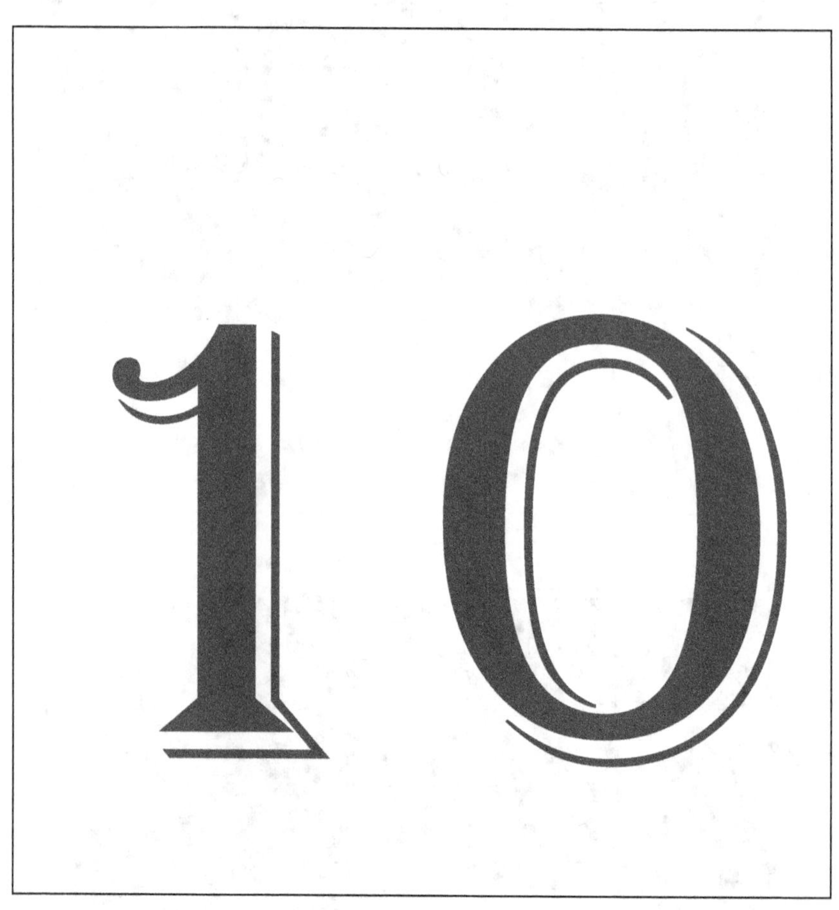

WALKING

With regards to work out, strolling is an optimal spot to begin. "Strolling is for all levels in the wellness venture. Strolling falls into the class of moderate-force high-impact practice when you stroll at a speed that stimulates your breathing to some degree

While does strolling qualify as an exercise as opposed to a couple of steps to a great extent to throw clothing in the dryer or get a nibble from the kitchen? like a 30-minute stroll through your area or a midday climb are significant for your general health.

Consider adding steps or slopes to your stroll to support the power.

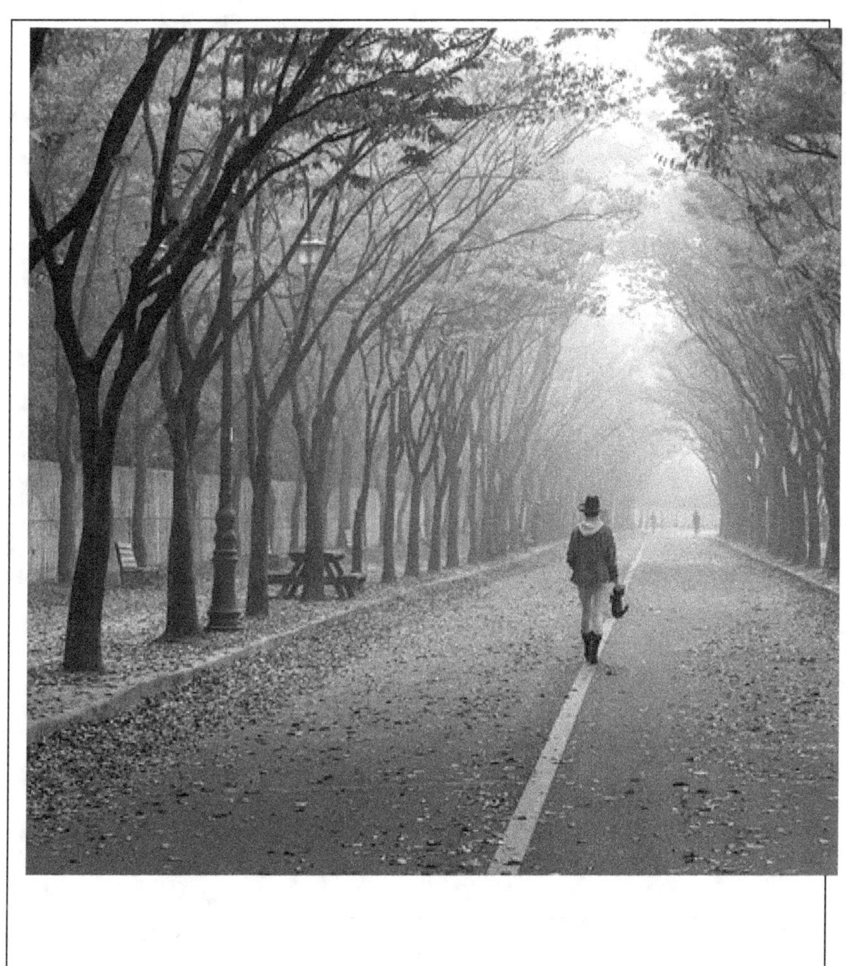

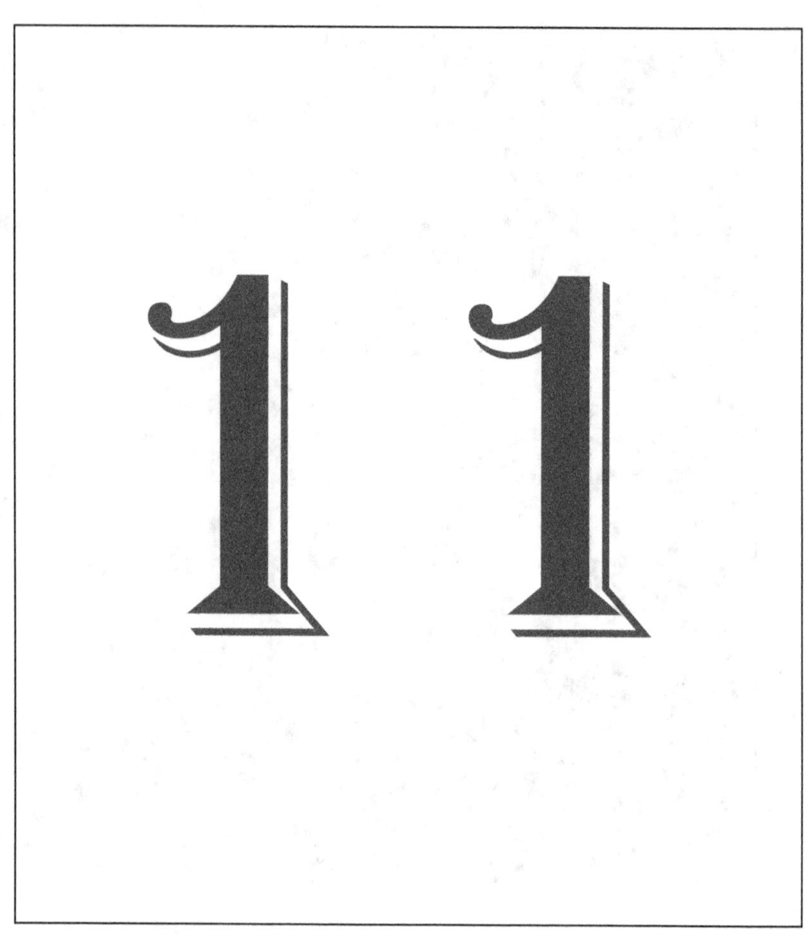

JUGGING

Jugging is a sort of running at a drowsy or loosened up pace. The essential objective is increment of health with less weight on the body than from faster running yet more than walking, or to save a steady speed for longer time periods. Go 30 minutes for each meeting. Allow no less than 8 to 12 weeks to advance toward ordinary running. Plan to broaden your running time each meeting, and switch between walking and running. Guarantee you warm up totally before you head out. Cool your body down with light stretches when you return.

Guarantee you have a great deal of fluids and take a water bottle with you on your run. Endeavor to hydrate already, during and after any activity.

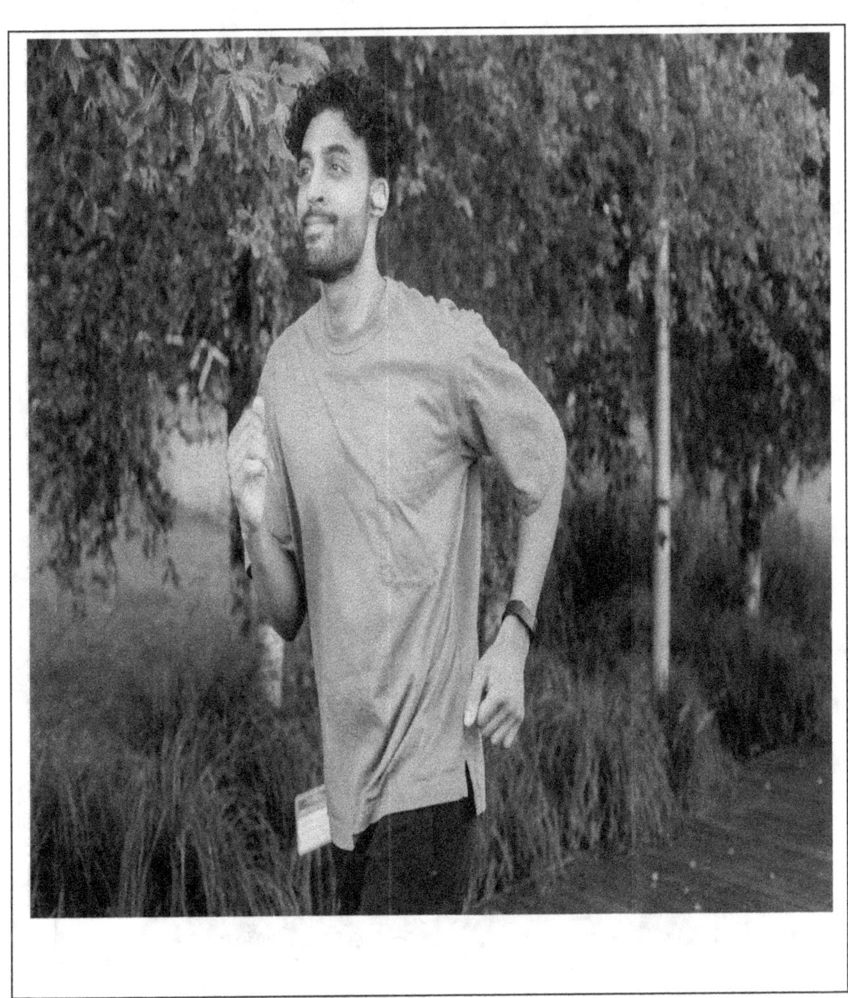

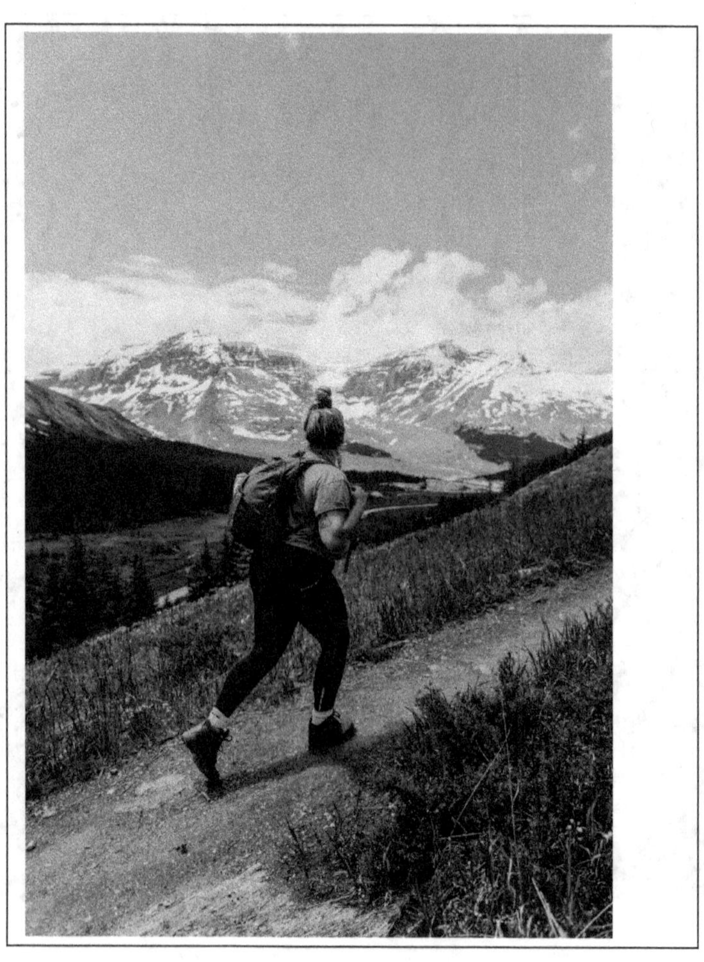

Create time for activities like swimming, playing soccer, playing football or playing basket ball. You can keep fit by doing something that would make you sweat by increasing your heart rate.

Your veins would open up and your heart can pump blood to your whole body keeping you refreshed.